SELF CARE AND STRESS MANAGEMENT

FOR NOVICES

Master The Art Of Balancing Life's Demands, Release Stress, Overcome Challenges, And Ignite Personal Growth With Proven Techniques For Wellness

DR. TADEO KASEN

Table of Contents

DISCLIAMER

This book is intended for informational and educational purposes only. The content provided in this book is not a substitute for professional medical advice, diagnosis, or treatment. Always seek the advice of your physician or other qualified health provider with any questions you may have regarding a medical condition.

The techniques and practices described in this book are based on general principles and may not be suitable for everyone. Individual results may vary, and it is important to consult with a qualified healthcare professional before undertaking any new health or wellness program.

The author and publisher of this book are not responsible for any adverse effects or consequences resulting from the use of information, suggestions, exercises, or techniques presented herein. The reader assumes full responsibility for his or her actions and choices. The information provided in this book is accurate and reliable. However, the author and publisher make no representation or warranties of any kind, express or implied, regarding the completeness, accuracy, reliability, or suitability of the information provided.

Any References to specific products, services, or organizations do not imply endorsement or recommendation by the author.

By reading this book, the reader acknowledges and agrees to the terms of this disclaimer. If the reader does not agree with these terms, they should not use the information provided in this book.

CHAPTER ONE

Introduction

Stress has become an unavoidable part of our everyday lives in our fast-paced and demanding environment. Stress, whether from jobs, relationships, or personal issues, may have an impact on both our physical and emotional health. To live a balanced and healthy life, it is important to acknowledge the importance of stress management and self-care routines.

Recognizing Stress

Stress is a normal reaction to stressful events, eliciting the body's "fight or flight" response. While short-term stress might be inspiring, long-term stress can be harmful to our health.

It can cause physical symptoms such as headaches, muscular tension, and exhaustion, as well as mental symptoms such as anxiety and irritation. Understanding the origins of stress is the first step toward successful stress management.

Work demands, financial difficulties, and relationship problems can all add to stress. Internal pressures such as negative self-talk or perfectionism can also be relevant. Recognizing stressors and their effects is essential for creating effective stress management techniques.

The Value Of Self-Care

Self-care is the deliberate and proactive activity of looking after one's physical, emotional, and mental health. It is not a luxury, but rather a must for general health and resilience in the face of stress. Individuals who ignore self-care become more vulnerable to the negative impacts of stress, which can lead to burnout and a drop in general well-being.

Prioritizing one's well-being is not selfish; it is an investment in one's ability to face life's obstacles. Setting boundaries, saying no when necessary, and making time for things that offer joy and relaxation are all part of it. Self-care activities develop a healthy relationship with oneself, fostering resilience and a better ability to manage stress.

Physical Self-Care Techniques

Physical self-care entails taking steps to preserve and improve one's body's health and vitality. These tactics not only improve general well-being but also help with stress management.

Exercise Regularly

Exercise is an excellent stress reducer. Endorphins, the body's natural mood boosters, are released, and stress hormone levels are reduced. Regular physical exercise, whether it's a brisk stroll, a gym workout, or a yoga session, is necessary for both physical and mental health.

Enough Sleep

A good night's sleep is essential for stress management. Sleep deprivation can worsen stress and impair the body's capacity to deal with obstacles. Establishing a consistent sleep schedule, maintaining a pleasant sleeping environment, and practicing relaxation methods before bedtime can all help you sleep better.

Healthy Eating

Another important part of physical self-care is eating a balanced and healthy diet. Nutrient-rich meals provide you the energy you need to deal with stress while limiting coffee, sugar, and processed foods can help you maintain a healthy mood and energy levels.

Techniques For Relaxation

Incorporating relaxation practices into everyday life can help to reduce physical stress and promote serenity. Deep breathing, progressive muscle relaxation, and mindfulness meditation are all techniques that may be used daily to reduce stress and improve general well-being.

Techniques For Emotional Self-Care

Emotional self-care is concerned with nourishing one's emotional well-being, cultivating resilience, and establishing appropriate coping skills.

Writing That Is Expressive

Writing about emotions and experiences may be a beneficial approach to process and release pent-up emotions. Individuals can obtain insights into their feelings and foster self-reflection by keeping a diary or engaging in expressive writing.

Make Contact With Others

Emotional well-being must establish and maintain strong social ties. Spending time with friends and family, discussing ideas and feelings, and seeking help when required may bring a sense of connection and comfort during difficult times.

Establish Limits

Setting and maintaining appropriate boundaries is an important element of emotional self-care. Learning to say no and prioritize one's needs can help prevent emotional tiredness and burnout.

Meditation And Mindfulness

Mindfulness and meditation can boost emotional resilience by encouraging present-moment awareness and acceptance. These techniques aid in the development of a nonjudgmental attitude toward one's thoughts and feelings, hence lowering tension and anxiety.

Finally, self-care and stress management are interwoven components of a comprehensive well-being strategy. Recognizing and comprehending stress, prioritizing self-care, and applying physical and emotional self-care practices are all important steps toward living a happier, more balanced life. Individuals may increase resilience, improve their capacity to cope with stress, and eventually improve their overall quality of life by doing these techniques.

Mental Self-Care Practices: Taking Care Of Your Inner World

It's easy to ignore the value of mental self-care in the hustle and bustle of daily living. This aspect of self-care is concerned with protecting and improving your psychological well-being. Incorporating mental self-care techniques into your routine is critical for keeping a healthy mind and handling life's problems.

Setting limits is a crucial mental self-care technique. Recognize your limitations and convey them effectively. Setting boundaries protects your mental health, whether it's saying no to extra work obligations, making time for personal activities, or creating a quiet area for introspection.

A positive outlook is another important part of mental self-care. Develop self-compassion and confront negative beliefs. Activities that offer you joy and laughter may improve your spirits and help you cope with the stresses of everyday life. Consider maintaining a thankfulness notebook to focus on the positive parts of your life, which will improve your general mental health.

Mindfulness techniques are also important for mental self-care. Being present in the moment, without judgment, is what mindfulness entails. Deep breathing, body scans, and guided meditation are all techniques that can help relieve tension and anxiety. Regular practice improves self-awareness, concentration, and emotional stability.

Finally, getting professional help is an important mental self-care activity. Having a focused area to examine your ideas and feelings, whether via therapy, counseling, or coaching, is critical for your mental well-being. Recognizing the need for outside assistance is a sign of strength, not weakness.

CHAPTER TWO

Relationships And Social Self-Care: Nurturing Connections

Humans are social creatures, and the quality of our interactions has a huge influence on our happiness. Social self-care entails developing meaningful connections, cultivating a feeling of belonging, and sustaining healthy relationships.

Setting and maintaining boundaries in your interactions is an important element of social self-care. Communicate your wants and expectations clearly while also respecting those of others. Healthy limits provide a positive environment that prevents fatigue and resentment.

Another important activity is making healthy social relationships. Surround yourself with people that raise you and encourage you. Nurturing healthy relationships, whether with family, friends, or coworkers, leads to a feeling of community and emotional well-being. Spend time doing things together, having meaningful talks, and celebrating each other's triumphs.

Social self-care, on the other hand, entails identifying poisonous connections and understanding when to let go. Consider reevaluating the importance of a relationship in your life if it constantly drains your energy, creates stress, or impedes your progress. Prioritize connections that are consistent with your ideals and contribute to your overall well-being.

Communication is the foundation of successful relationships, and active listening is a skill that should be honed. Give people your undivided attention, convey empathy, and affirm their sentiments. Building trust and open communication leads to stronger ties and a more supportive social network.

Finally, remember to include time for self-reflection in your social self-care practice. Examine the dynamics of your relationships, look for trends, and make deliberate decisions about who you want to invest your time and energy in. Healthy, meaningful relationships make a substantial contribution to your overall happiness and resilience.

Making A Self-Care Strategy: Intentional Well-Being

Making a self-care strategy is akin to creating a road map to happiness. It entails making deliberate, proactive efforts to prioritize your physical, emotional, and mental wellness. A tailored self-care strategy is vital for managing life's challenges and sustaining long-term balance.

Begin by determining your unique requirements and priorities. Consider the various components of well-being, such as physical, emotional, mental, social, and spiritual well-being. Consider what hobbies and behaviors offer you joy, relaxation, and contentment.

Create a realistic and doable strategy after you've established your self-care priorities. Break down more ambitious goals into more manageable chores.

For example, if physical activity is important to you, create a weekly workout regimen that fits within your schedule. If relaxing is a priority, plan regular pauses or moments of awareness throughout the day.

Implementing a self-care strategy requires consistency. Include self-care activities in your daily, weekly, and monthly schedules. Self-care should be treated as a non-negotiable component of your calendar, just like work or other obligations. This deliberate approach guarantees that self-care becomes a long-term and essential component of your lifestyle.

Reassess and adapt your self-care strategy regularly as your needs and circumstances change. Life is ever-changing, and so should your self-care routine. Depending on your present position, be open to exploring new activities or modifying the frequency and intensity of existing ones.

Remember that self-care is not selfish; it is an essential investment in your health. Prioritizing yourself helps you to completely participate in other aspects of your life, such as relationships, employment, or personal activities. You are taking proactive control of your health and happiness by developing and implementing a self-care strategy.

Cultivating Present Awareness Through Mindfulness And Meditation

Mindfulness and meditation are effective techniques for stress management and overall well-being. These practices, which have their roots in ancient traditions, have earned global attention for their good influence on mental and emotional health.

Mindfulness entails paying conscious attention to the current moment without judgment. It is about becoming more aware of your thoughts, feelings, and environment.

Regular mindfulness practice can help to reduce stress, anxiety, and rumination while improving attention, resilience, and emotional control.

Meditation is a type of mindfulness practice that often includes concentrated attention, deep breathing, and guided imagery. Mindfulness meditation, loving-kindness meditation, and body scan meditation are examples of meditation approaches. Find a style that appeals to you and implement it into your daily routine.

To begin, set aside a few minutes each day to focus on your breath or notice your thoughts without becoming embroiled in them. Increase the length gradually as you get more comfortable with the practice. Consider utilizing meditation apps or going to guided sessions to help you along your journey.

Mindfulness is not restricted to formal meditation; it may be integrated into daily activities as well. Practice mindful dining by savoring each mouthful, mindful walking by focusing on each step, or focused listening in talks. These modest moments of present awareness add up to a more attentive and grounded life.

Mindfulness and meditation have more advantages than just stress reduction. They can improve cognitive skills, boost emotional well-being, and build a stronger sense of self and others. As you include mindfulness in your everyday routine, you will most certainly notice an increase in your general quality of life.

Habits Of A Healthy Lifestyle: Nourishing Your Body And Mind

A healthy lifestyle, which includes physical, mental, and emotional elements, is the cornerstone of well-being. Positive behaviors improve your general resilience and capacity to cope with stress. Here are some fundamental elements of a healthy lifestyle:

1. Regular Exercise: Physical activity is not only important for maintaining a healthy weight, but it also helps to reduce stress, improve mood, and improve cognitive performance. Find activities that you love, such as walking, running, yoga, or dancing, and include them in your daily routine.

2. Balanced Nutrition: A well-rounded, healthy diet is vital for both physical and mental wellness. Give emphasis on whole foods, such as whole grains, lean meats, and fruits and vegetables. Stay hydrated and watch your dietary habits, striving for a balanced and long-term strategy.

3. Quality Sleep: Adequate and restful sleep is critical for overall health. Establish a consistent sleep regimen, make your sleeping environment pleasant, and emphasize obtaining the necessary amount of sleep each night. Sleep is associated with increased mood, cognitive performance, and stress resilience.

4. Stress Management approaches: Aside from mindfulness and meditation, investigate alternative stress management approaches. This might include gradual muscular relaxation, deep breathing techniques, or indulging in relaxing activities. Try several things to see what works best for you.

5. Time Management: Managing your time well helps to a sense of control and minimizes stress. Set realistic objectives, prioritize work, and divide bigger projects into smaller, achievable phases. When feasible, learn to delegate and realize the value of downtime in preserving overall balance.

6. Hydration: Staying hydrated is essential for physical and mental health. Water is necessary for several body activities, including digestion, circulation, and temperature control. Make it a habit to drink water throughout the day to improve your overall health.

7. Social Connections: Healthy connections are not only an important element of social self-care, but they are also essential to living a healthy lifestyle. Positive social ties give emotional support, minimize feelings of isolation, and increase overall life satisfaction.

8. Continuous Learning and Growth: Mental health must engage in activities that excite the mind and foster personal growth. Continuous learning, whether by reading, attending classes, or engaging in hobbies, develops a sense of purpose and fulfillment.

CHAPTER THREE

Holistic Self-Care For A Healthy Lifestyle

Incorporating mental self-care activities, cultivating social relationships, developing a tailored self-care plan, embracing mindfulness and meditation, and adopting healthy lifestyle choices all contribute to a holistic well-being approach. Recognizing the interdependence of physical, mental, and emotional health enables you to build resilience and more easily overcome life's obstacles.

Self-care is a dynamic and individualized journey, not a one-size-fits-all idea. Experiment with various methods, be gentle with yourself and modify your self-care regimen as required.

Self-care is an investment in your general health, happiness, and capacity to live a happy life. Remember that self-care is not a luxury; it is a must for a healthy and happy life.

Stress Reduction Through Time Management

Amid the rush and bustle of everyday life, time management is critical to maintaining a healthy balance and lowering stress. Effective time management helps you to prioritize work, utilize resources appropriately, and gain control over your calendar. Here are some time management ideas to add to your routine for stress reduction:

1. Prioritize Tasks: Identify and prioritize your tasks based on their significance and urgency. To-do lists and productivity apps can help you plan your day. This aids in dividing large jobs into manageable chunks, lowering stress linked with the sense of being overwhelmed.

2. Set Realistic Goals: Be realistic about your ability to complete tasks in a given period. Setting unreasonable expectations might result in dissatisfaction and increased stress. Break down huge goals into smaller, more manageable tasks, and celebrate each milestone's fulfillment.

3. Avoid multitasking: While it may appear to be an effective approach to getting more done, it frequently leads to lower productivity and greater stress.

Concentrate on one activity at a time and give it your undivided attention before moving on to the next. This improves productivity while also reducing the mental strain involved with juggling many jobs.

4. Recognize your limitations and don't be afraid to deny new duties when you're feeling overwhelmed. Saying no is not a sign of weakness; it is a necessary ability for achieving a good work-life balance.

5. Delegate chores: If at all practicable, delegate chores to others. Delegating not only reduces your burden but also promotes collaboration. It is critical to delegate work to others so that you may focus on things that need your particular talents and knowledge.

6. Time Blocking: Assign specified blocks of time to certain tasks. For example, set aside some hours for work, others for personal hobbies, and make time for leisure. This methodical technique aids in striking a balance between work and personal life.

7. Limit Distractions: Recognize and reduce sources of distraction. To secure your concentrated work time, turn off non-essential alerts, create a quiet workstation, and set boundaries. By reducing distractions, you improve your capacity to focus on the work at hand.

8. Regular breaks are necessary for sustaining productivity and minimizing stress. Include brief rest and recharge intervals throughout the day. Make use of this time to stretch, go for a stroll, or indulge in things that offer you joy and relaxation.

You may create a more ordered and controlled environment by applying these time management tactics, thereby lowering stress and fostering a better lifestyle.

Creating Limits

Setting and keeping clear boundaries is critical for effective stress management. Boundaries establish your willingness and ability to accomplish things, laying the groundwork for good relationships and work-life balance. When establishing limits, keep the following points in mind:

1. Define Your Limits: Recognize your physical, emotional, and mental boundaries. Recognizing these boundaries is the first step toward putting effective time, energy, and commitment restrictions in place.

2. Communicate Openly: Make your limits clear to others. This includes coworkers, friends, and family members. When stating your requirements and restrictions, be aggressive yet courteous. Effective communication ensures that your expectations are understood by others and helps to avoid misunderstandings.

3. Learn to Say No: The ability to say no is a powerful and vital talent. Requests or obligations that surpass your present capabilities or jeopardize your well-being should be politely declined. Saying no is not a rejection, but rather a deliberate decision to safeguard your time and energy.

4. Make Self-Care a Priority: Make self-care a non-negotiable element of your routine. This involves making time for things that will revitalize and nurture your mind and body. Making self-care a priority promotes the value of your well-being and establishes a precedent for others to respect your personal space.

5. Establish job-life Boundaries: In this day and age, it is critical to distinguish between job and personal life. Define work hours clearly and avoid performing job-related things outside of these periods. To maintain a good work-life balance, disconnect from business emails and phone calls during personal time.

6. Connections: Consider the influence of your connections on your overall well-being. Be in the company of individuals who respect and acknowledge your boundaries. If particular connections repeatedly test your boundaries, consider setting stricter boundaries or reevaluating the relationship.

7. Maintain Consistency: Maintaining boundaries requires consistency. Respect your boundaries once you've set them. This constancy emphasizes the value of limits to both yourself and those around you.

8. Reassess and Adjust: Reassess your boundaries regularly, especially during substantial life changes or times of high stress. As your objectives and capacities change, you may need to make changes. Setting and changing limits with flexibility is critical for long-term stress management.

Setting and maintaining boundaries is a proactive stress-reduction strategy. It gives you the ability to take charge of your time, energy, and relationships, resulting in a happier and more balanced life.

Seeking Assistance

When you have a solid support system, navigating life's problems becomes easier. Seeking help is an important part of stress management since it provides emotional, practical, and social support. Here are some strategies for efficiently seeking and utilizing assistance:

1. Identify Your Needs: Determine your unique assistance requirements. Knowing what you need, whether it's emotional support, practical aid, or someone to listen, allows you to communicate successfully with possible allies.

2. Communicate Openly: Express your thoughts and needs to friends, family, and coworkers. Effective communication is the cornerstone for obtaining the assistance you need. Be open about your difficulties and let others know how they may help.

3. Create a diversified supporting Network: Create a diversified network of supporting individuals. This includes friends, family members, mentors, and coworkers. Having a diverse support system guarantees that you may seek assistance from a variety of sources.

4. Consider obtaining expert assistance as necessary. Therapists, counselors, and support groups can provide professional help for specific difficulties such as mental health issues, grieving, or marital problems. Professional assistance can give useful insights and coping skills.

5. Join Supportive Communities: Connect with people who share your interests or problems. Support groups, whether online or in person, provide a sense of connection and understanding. Connecting with those who have been in similar situations may give empathy as well as practical assistance.

6. When you're feeling overwhelmed, don't be afraid to assign duties or obligations. Seek assistance from

family members, friends, or coworkers. Sharing responsibilities not only lightens the strain but also develops relationships.

7. Be Receptive to Reciprocity: Help is a two-way street. Always be willing to lend a hand to those in need.   Creating a mutually helpful network strengthens ties and builds a feeling of community.

8. Self-advocacy is the act of advocating for one's own needs. Communicate clearly how people can help you, whether via active listening, practical aid, or company. Being proactive in getting help allows you to deal with difficulties more successfully.

Seeking help is not a sign of weakness but of strength and self-awareness. Accepting help from others improves your capacity to handle problems and increases overall well-being.

Relaxation Techniques: In today's fast-paced world, relaxation techniques have become crucial tools for stress management and general well-being. These techniques try to trigger the body's natural relaxation response, therefore mitigating the detrimental consequences of chronic stress. Deep breathing exercises, gradual muscular relaxation, and guided visualization are all excellent relaxation strategies. Individuals can relieve stress and achieve inner calm by focusing on their breath or methodically relaxing muscular regions.

Incorporating mindfulness meditation and yoga into everyday activities promotes relaxation while also improving mental and physical resilience. Regular use of these techniques not only decreases stress but also improves sleep quality, mood, and focus, all of which contribute to a more balanced and meaningful existence.

Gratitude and Positive Thinking: Practicing gratitude and positive thinking is a great stress management and mental-well-being practice. Gratitude entails recognizing and appreciating the wonderful parts of life, especially when faced with difficulties. Keeping a gratitude diary, in which people routinely jot down things they are grateful for, can help people shift their focus away from stressors and foster a good outlook. Positive thinking entails reframing negative thoughts and establishing a positive attitude. Recognizing and correcting negative self-talk can reduce stress dramatically. Practicing self-compassion and concentrating on one's strengths and accomplishments also lead to a more resilient mentality. According to research, people who practice gratitude and positive thinking have lower stress levels, better emotional health, and a higher overall feeling of life satisfaction. Incorporating these strategies into daily life has the potential to be transformative, fostering a more balanced and constructive attitude to stress management.

CHAPTER FOUR

Hobbies And Recreation For Stress Reduction

Finding time for hobbies and recreation may appear to be a luxury in the rush and bustle of modern life, but it is an important element of self-care and stress management. Participating in activities that you like not only gives you a vacation from daily stresses but also helps your general well-being.

Hobbies can range from creative endeavors like painting or playing an instrument to physical ones like hiking, gardening, or sports. The goal is to choose hobbies that make you happy and give you a sense of achievement. These pleasurable experiences serve as a counterpoint to the pressures in your life, helping you to refuel and confront difficulties with renewed vigor.

Recreation, on the other hand, entails deliberate downtime. This might be as easy as reading a book, going for a leisurely walk, or spending time with family and friends. The idea is to participate in activities that allow you to unwind and detach from work or other sources of stress. It's all about allowing your mind to reset before returning to your obligations with a fresh perspective.

A proactive strategy for stress management is to incorporate hobbies and entertainment into your routine. Making time for activities you like not only reduces stress in the present but also creates a reservoir of pleasant memories to draw on during difficult times. This investment in your well-being will pay off in terms of general mental and emotional resilience.

Stress Reduction Through Sleep Hygiene

Quality sleep is essential for overall health and stress management. Despite this, many people in our fast-paced culture deal with sleep-related disorders. Establishing appropriate sleep hygiene habits is critical for getting enough rest and improving your capacity to cope with stress.

Adopting routines and behaviors that promote consistent and restful sleep is what sleep hygiene entails. Maintaining a regular sleep schedule, providing a pleasant sleep environment, and avoiding stimulants such as caffeine or electronic gadgets close to bedtime are all part of this. The idea is to tell your body and mind that it's time to unwind and prepare for sleep.

Sleep deprivation not only lowers cognitive function but also raises stress levels. Chronic sleep deprivation can lead to depression, anxiety, and a compromised immune system. Prioritizing sleep is a type of self-care that has a direct influence on your capacity to deal with life's obstacles.

Creating a peaceful and clutter-free sleep environment, establishing a nighttime ritual, and reducing lights before sleep are all important stages in improving sleep hygiene. Additionally, minimizing blue-light exposure on screens and avoiding large meals close to bedtime help to improve sleep quality.

Recognizing the significance of sleep and taking action to enhance sleep hygiene is a proactive stress management method. By giving your body and mind the rest they require, you can handle life's stresses with more resilience and clarity.

Stress Reduction Nutrition

The connection between diet and stress management is complex and frequently overlooked. What you eat has a direct influence on your energy levels, emotions, and general health. Adopting a healthy, balanced diet is an important component of self-care that adds to your capacity to deal with stress successfully.

Certain diets, including those high in omega-3 fatty acids, antioxidants, and complex carbohydrates, have been associated with better mood and stress resilience.

Excessive consumption of processed foods, sweets, and caffeine, on the other hand, might add to feelings of worry and exhaustion.

Eating a range of nutrient-dense meals gives your body the building blocks it needs for optimal operation. Fruits, vegetables, and whole grains, which are high in vitamins and minerals, benefit both your physical and mental health. Adequate water is also essential since dehydration can cause weariness and increased stress.

Mindful eating, paying attention to hunger and fullness cues, and avoiding emotional eating are all important practices for a healthy relationship with food. Creating a healthy link between diet and well-being is a proactive step toward stress management.

Exercise And Stress Reduction

Physical activity is a strong stress-relieving and general well-being strategy. Regular exercise has been demonstrated to lower anxiety and depression symptoms while also boosting mood and cognitive performance. Exercise, whether it's a brisk stroll, a yoga session, or a full-fledged workout, is a proactive approach to stress management.

Endorphins, the body's natural mood boosters, are released during exercise, generating a sensation of well-being. Furthermore, physical exercise releases pent-up energy and tension, aiding in the reduction of the physiological consequences of stress on the body.

Personal preferences and physical conditions might influence the type and intensity of exercise. Finding things that you like and that fit into your schedule are the key. Because consistency is more essential than intensity, even brief bouts of exercise regularly can have a major influence on stress reduction.

Including physical activity in your regular routine doesn't have to be tough. It may be as easy as taking the stairs instead of the elevator, going for a stroll during your lunch break, or doing a fast home exercise. The idea is to include exercise in your daily routine, which will improve your physical and mental resilience.

Work And Personal Life Balance

In today's fast-paced world, striking a balance between work and personal life is a constant challenge. Finding this balance, on the other hand, is critical for general well-being and successful stress management. Work-life balance improves job happiness, decreases burnout, and adds to a more meaningful personal life.

It is critical to establish clear boundaries between work and personal time. This involves setting clear work hours, resisting the need to bring work home, and unplugging from business-related interactions during personal time. Setting these limits helps to keep the distinctions between business and personal life from merging.

Another important aspect of finding balance is effective time management. Setting realistic objectives, prioritizing chores, and learning to delegate when required are all abilities that contribute to a more manageable burden.

Maintaining a good work-life balance is a continuous process that needs constant observation and modification.

Breaks and holidays are essential for recharging and avoiding burnout. Stepping away from work helps you to unwind, indulge in enjoyable hobbies, and spend valuable time with loved ones. It's not only self-care, but it's also an investment in your long-term productivity and well-being.

CHAPTER FIVE

Adapting To Change

Change is an unavoidable aspect of life, and understanding how to deal with it is critical for stress management. Whether it's a large life shift like a job move or relocation, or a smaller, everyday adjustment, adapting to new circumstances necessitates resilience and coping abilities.

Maintaining a positive outlook is an important strategy for dealing with change. Adopting a growth-oriented mindset helps you to perceive change as a source of personal and professional improvement rather than a danger. Flexibility and adaptability serve to ease the transition and lessen the stress associated with the uncertainty.

Creating a support network is critical during times of transition. Having a network of people you can turn to for advice and emotional support, whether it's friends, family, or coworkers, offers a sense of security. Communicating freely about your thoughts and receiving advice from individuals who have gone through similar transitions may be quite beneficial.

Taking care of your physical and emotional health is especially crucial during times of transition. Prioritizing self-care activities such as exercise, appropriate sleep, and relaxation methods can help you retain your resilience and manage the challenges that come with transition.

Building Resilience

Resilience is the capacity to recover from misfortune and face obstacles with a positive attitude. It's a trait that may be developed through a variety of activities and attitude modifications. Building resilience is a proactive strategy for stress management that will better equip you to confront life's uncertainties.

Developing a development mindset is a critical component of resilience. Accepting adversities as opportunities for personal growth and learning rather than as insurmountable hurdles promotes resilience.

This shift in viewpoint helps you to tackle problems with interest and drive.

Another important component in developing resilience is the development of strong social ties. Having a support network of friends, family, and coworkers gives emotional support and a variety of opinions during difficult times. Sharing your experiences and listening to others' tales strengthens your feeling of community and your ability to overcome obstacles.

Mindfulness and stress reduction strategies, such as meditation and deep breathing exercises, promote emotional control and reduce the physiological impacts of stress, which contribute to resilience. These activities assist you in remaining grounded and focused in the face of hardship.

Managing Burnout

Burnout is a widespread problem in today's demanding workplace, defined by persistent working stress that has not been effectively controlled.

Coping with burnout necessitates a multifaceted strategy that tackles both the underlying reasons for weariness and disengagement.

Recognizing the presence of burnout is one of the first stages in dealing with it. Recognizing the indicators of burnout, such as emotional tiredness, decreased performance, and a sense of detachment, helps you to take preventative actions before the condition becomes incapacitating.

Setting realistic limits and learning to say no are important skills for avoiding and managing burnout. Prioritizing self-care, delegating responsibilities when appropriate, and communicating honestly with supervisors and coworkers about workload and expectations are all critical.

Regular pauses, both during the day and on holidays, are critical for avoiding burnout. Hobbies and spending time with loved ones are examples of activities that can replenish your physical and emotional reserves.

Seeking professional assistance, such as counseling or therapy, is an important step in dealing with burnout. Speaking with a mental health professional provides a safe environment to investigate the root reasons for burnout, develop coping techniques, and strive toward a healthy work-life balance.

Professional Assistance And Counseling

While self-care practices are beneficial, there are occasions when professional assistance and therapy are required for successful stress management. When dealing with chronic stress, mental health issues, or big life transitions, seeking the advice of a skilled expert may make a tremendous impact on your overall well-being.

Counseling provides a safe and supportive environment in which to examine your ideas, feelings, and actions. A counselor can assist you in gaining insights into the core causes of stress, developing coping methods, and working toward good life changes.

Individual requirements and the unique difficulties being addressed dictate the therapeutic method. CBT, for example, focuses on modifying negative thinking patterns and behaviors, whereas mindfulness-based treatments encourage present-moment awareness and stress reduction.

In circumstances when there is a considerable influence on mental health, medication may be advised. Psychiatric doctors can determine if medication is an appropriate treatment choice and track its success in conjunction with counseling.

Seeking professional treatment is a proactive step in prioritizing your mental health. It exhibits self-awareness and a willingness to face obstacles constructively and helpfully. A mental health expert can provide you with the tools and methods you need for stress management and general well-being.

Finally, self-care and stress management are complicated ideas that need a comprehensive approach.

A comprehensive stress management strategy includes incorporating hobbies and recreation, maintaining good sleep hygiene, prioritizing nutrition, engaging in regular exercise, balancing work and personal life, coping with change, building resilience, addressing burnout, and seeking professional help when needed.

Individuals may improve their well-being, build resilience, and negotiate life's obstacles more easily by proactively applying these tactics.

Conclusion On Self-Care And Stress Management

To summarize, practicing self-care and stress management is not a luxury but a vital requirement for general well-being.

As people manage the complexity of contemporary life, prioritizing self-care becomes increasingly important in minimizing the negative consequences of stress. The path to good health is a multifaceted strategy that includes physical, mental, and emotional aspects.

Individuals empower themselves to cope with life's obstacles more successfully by adopting self-care techniques into daily routines continuously. Engaging in mindfulness exercises, regular exercise, appropriate sleep, or developing meaningful connections all lead to resilience and a better capacity to deal with challenges.

Furthermore, it is critical to recognize that self-care is not a one-size-fits-all idea. Each person's self-care regimen must be tailored to their specific requirements and preferences. This tailored strategy improves the long-term viability and efficacy of stress management measures.

Finally, the benefits of self-care go beyond personal well-being, favorably impacting relationships, job productivity, and society dynamics.

Adopting the notion that self-care is a proactive investment in one's health supports a resilient culture and a healthier, more balanced society as a whole.

In this sense, self-care and stress management are not just acts of self-love, but also a societal obligation for a more peaceful and robust society.